D1736739

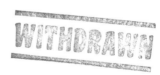

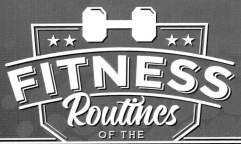

SIMONE BILES

Fitness Routines OF THE SUPERSTAR ATHLETES

JEFF SAVAGE

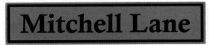

Mitchell Lane
PUBLISHERS

2001 SW 31st Avenue
Hallandale, FL 33009

www.mitchelllane.com

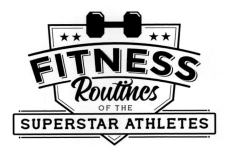

First Edition, 2020.
Author: Jeff Savage
Designer: Ed Morgan
Editor: Lisa Petrillo

Series: Fitness Routines of the Superstar Athletes
Title: Simone Biles / by Jeff Savage

Hallandale, FL : Mitchell Lane Publishers, [2020]

Library bound ISBN: 9781680204599
eBook ISBN: 9781680204605

Contents

Chapter ONE
Back on Top..4

Chapter TWO
Pure Gold.. 8

Chapter THREE
Fitness Force..14

Chapter FOUR
Nutrition and Focus....................................22

Chapter FIVE
Commitment..26

Awards..28
Timeline..29
Glossary.. 30
Further Reading...31
On the Internet..31
Index.. 32
About the Author.......................................32

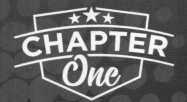
BACK ON *Top*

Simone Biles was all smiles. She was
competing in the 2018 U.S. Classic—
an important national gymnastics meet.
After two events, Biles was in first place.
She had dazzled the crowd in Columbus,
Ohio, with an acrobatic **floor routine** and a
soaring **vault** where she seemed to fall
straight out of the sky.

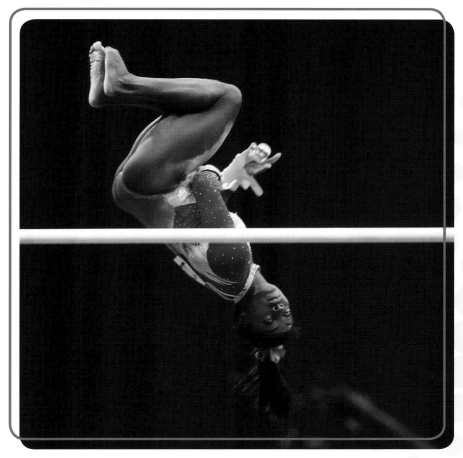

Simone Biles competes on the uneven bars during the U.S. Classic gymnastics event in July 2018.

Moments later, her smile was gone. On the **uneven bars**, Biles reached short on a move and dropped from the bar. The mistake was costly. She recovered to complete her routine cleanly. But her lower score left her in second place overall. She had one event left.

Chapter ONE

Second place is normally a fine result. Not for Simone Biles. She hadn't lost an all-around competition in five years. In that time, she had become the most decorated American gymnast ever. Her last competition before this was her greatest—the 2016 Olympic Games in Rio de Janeiro, Brazil, where she won a record four gold medals. But that was more than two years ago. Biles hadn't competed since.

Teenagers dominate women's gymnastics at the **elite level**. In the last 40 years, every all-around Olympic champion has been a teen. When Biles performed her magic at the Rio Games she was 19 years old, second oldest of all the winners (by four days). That's the age when gymnastics careers normally come to an end. Yet here she was, two years later, at the "old" age of 21, still competing and expecting to win. How was this possible?

Biles competes in the floor exercise.

6

Biles was often as giggly as a pre-teen. But right now she was serious, mad even, her sights fixed on her final event—the **balance beam**. She needed a solid score of 14.00 to retake first place. Her two-minute performance was nearly flawless. She spun three circles from a **squat** to show her power. She did a front flip with a half turn and another in the **pike** position. She did a back handspring to two back **layouts**. She dismounted with a double back handspring full-rotation double somersault. She stuck the landing and raised her arms skyward. Her 15.20 score was the highest of the event. Her 58.70 total was the best overall score all year. Her smile returned.

Biles described her attitude to the media afterward, saying, "I was like, 'You know what, Simone? Just forget about bars and go do a nice clean beam routine.' I was pretty proud of how I handled it. I think this is a good starting point. There's still a lot to work on. But we're in a pretty good place."

Fun Fact

In 2016 Biles was named one of the Most Influential People in the World listed by *TIME* magazine.

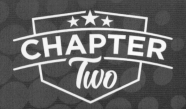

PURE
Gold

Simone Arianne Biles was born March 14, 1997, in Columbus, Ohio. She was the third of four children born to Shanon Biles. Simone never knew her birth father. Shanon was addicted to drugs and alcohol and unable to care for her children. Simone was 3 when she and her younger sister, Adria, were sent to live with her grandparents in Spring, Texas. Simone's grandparents—Ron and Nellie Biles— adopted the young girls to become their legal parents. "When we came down, it was automatically, 'OK, you're my mom and you're my dad,'" Simone told a reporter. "There was never a question about it."

Biles competes at the 2013 World Gymnastics Championships in Belgium.

As a child, Simone jumped from bed to bed and did flips on the couch, and at age 6, her parents enrolled her in gymnastics classes Bannon's Gymnastix. Two years later she started training with coach Aimee Boorman and slowly rose through the junior ranks. With the senior and elite levels within reach, she faced a decision: attend the public high school with her friends, or be home-schooled so she could practice more hours. She chose home schooling. She won the all-around national title and then the 2013 World Gymnastics Championships in Belgium. She won the world title again in 2014 in China and a third time in 2015 in Scotland to become the first female in history to win three straight world all-around titles.

Chapter TWO

Biles was at the top of her sport when she arrived in Rio for the Olympic Games. She won gold medals in the team competition and the individual vault, floor exercise, and all-around, setting a U.S. record for most gold medals at a single Games. Many were calling her the greatest gymnast ever.

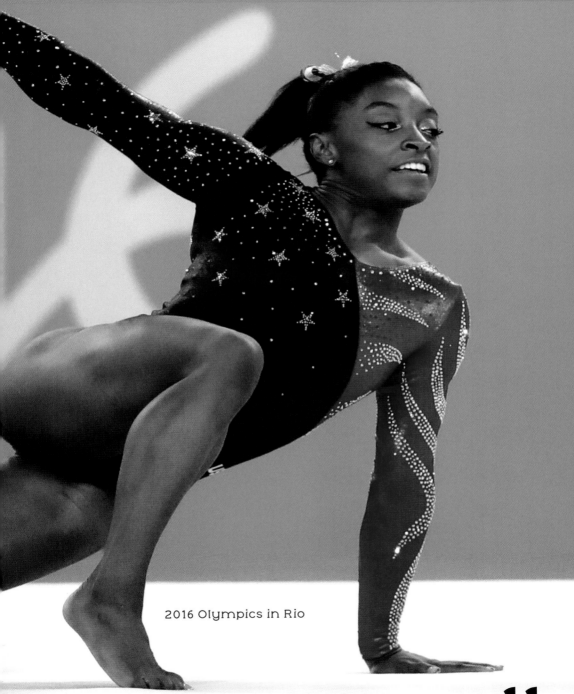

2016 Olympics in Rio

Following the Olympics, Biles left gymnastics. She spent more than a year traveling to such places as Belize, Hawaii, London, and Monte Carlo. Back home, she helped write a book that became a made-for-TV movie. She competed on the television show *Dancing With the Stars*. She made commercials for several companies and her face appeared on billboards and advertising posters. "Whenever we passed one at the airport, my mom was like, 'Simone, go stand next to it, so I can take a picture,'" said Biles. "And I was like, 'Mommmm, we've already seen all of them.'"

Biles turned 21 years old in 2018. She was a millionaire. It seemed logical that her gymnastics career had ended. Instead, she was back in the gym, training as hard as ever. She was preparing for the 2020 Olympics in Tokyo, Japan. She wanted to become the first woman to repeat as all-around champion in more than half a century. She would also be the *oldest* to do so. She says she is on her way. "The 2018 Simone," she declared to reporters, "is better than the 2016 Simone."

Fun Fact

At the Rio Olympics, Biles was chosen as the Team USA flag bearer for the closing ceremony. She carried the American flag as she led more than 500 U.S. athletes into the stadium.

13

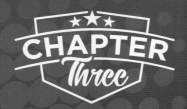

FITNESS
Force

The Olympic motto is *Faster, Higher, Stronger.* It was created in 1894. But it's almost as if the phrase was written with Simone Biles in mind. Her blurring sprints down the runway, high-flying aerobatics, and dynamic skills are unmatched on the planet.

Biles is just 4 feet, 8 inches in height. Of the 555 athletes who represented the United States at the Rio Olympics, Biles was the shortest of all. Her small frame is a disadvantage in gymnastics. The distance between the uneven bars for her is greater. Her tiny hands make it hard to grip the bars. Biles overcomes her shortness with sheer strength. "She is the greatest gymnast ever, the best I've ever seen in my life," Mary Lou Retton told a magazine writer. Retton was the first American woman to win the individual all-around Olympic gold medal, back in 1984. "A lot of us athletes and Olympic champions joke that she's so strong she should have to compete with the men. She's that strong."

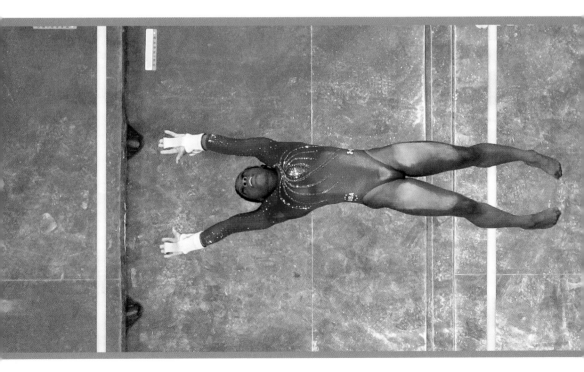

Biles competes on the uneven bars during the women's U.S. Olympic gymnastics trials July 2016.

Biles has developed her powerhouse body with a grueling fitness routine. At the junior level, she worked out 20 hours a week. At age 14 she ramped up to 32 hours a week—twice a day on weekdays and once on Saturday. Resuming training for the 2020 Olympics, she added even more hours to her fitness program. She trains at the World Champions Centre in her hometown of Spring. Her parents built the training center in 2014.

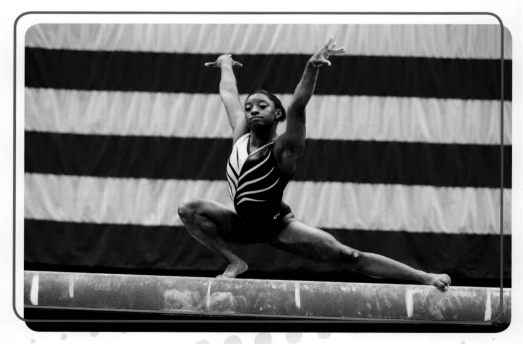

Training at the World Champions Centre in 2014

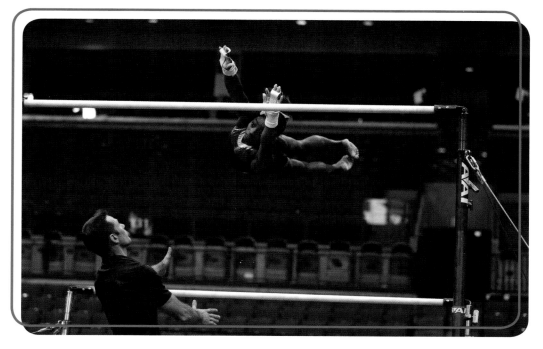

Training with Laurent Landi

Biles spends most morning sessions working on basics and skills. New coach Laurent Landi makes sure her arms, legs, feet, and body are positioned properly. In the afternoon, Biles puts skill sets together that she worked on that morning. She focuses often on practicing on the beam and bars. Sometimes she concentrates on a single move, such as a tumbling run featuring a double layout with a half twist. Biles created this move, and so it is known as the "Biles." As a competition nears, Biles works on pressure sets, in which she performs her entire routine as if the judges are there.

Biles develops power with strength training. She performs daily whole-body routines, meaning she trains every body part every day. She does exercises for her lower body, core (the body's midsection), and upper body. Biles prefers lower body work. She doesn't like exercising her core but admits it is the most important area to train.

Biles generates explosive force with her legs. Her sturdy lower body also protects her from injury after thousands of hard landings, year after year. She does mainly bodyweight exercises such as **lunges**, front squats, and jump squats.

A solid core provides strength and helps prevent injury. Biles says she would rather strengthen her core by laughing. Instead, she does exercises such as **crunches**, **planks**, and leg raises hanging from a wall ladder.

Biles trains so hard to be the best that since age 14, she has worked out 32 hours a week.

Biles has a strong upper body. She can pull herself up a 20-foot climbing rope in six seconds! Her wide shoulders and muscled arms lift her on bars and propel her off vault. What does Biles do to strengthen her upper body? She likes chin-ups, pull-ups, and especially handstand pushups.

Cross training is participating in a sport other than the athlete's usual sport. Biles has cross-trained using the events of a **triathlon**. She swam twice weekly—almost a mile each time. She biked 10 miles. She ran a mile and went straight to the beam to perform a routine.

Biles spends a lot of time after a workout stretching her muscles. Stretching keeps her flexible, reduces tension, and helps prevent injury. Her favorite stretch is splits because they're easy for her. She likes over-splits, in which she puts one leg up on a mat so it's higher, because, as she told a reporter, "It just looks cooler!"

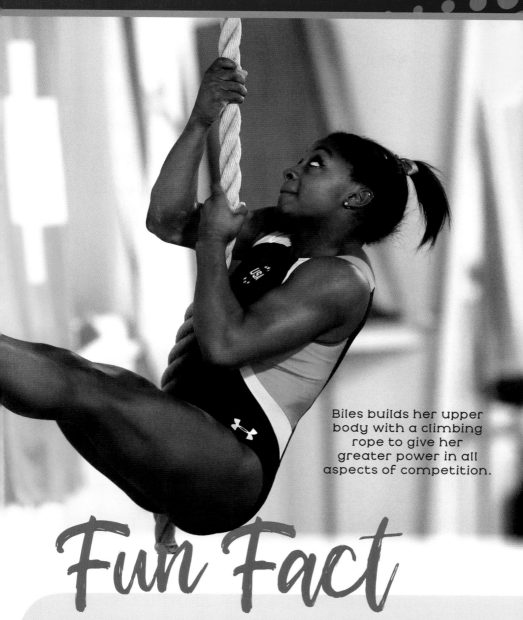

Biles builds her upper body with a climbing rope to give her greater power in all aspects of competition.

Fun Fact

Simone's family has four pet German Shepherds, and a turtle collection for good luck.

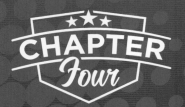

CHAPTER *Four*

NUTRITION and *Focus*

Working out more than 30 hours a week takes lots of energy. Food is energy. Biles fuels her body with healthy foods.

For breakfast she eats egg whites for protein and cereal and fruit for carbohydrates. After a workout she drinks a protein shake and eats a banana and peanut butter. The potassium in a banana reduces muscle cramps. For lunch she eats chicken or fish. For dinner she likes salmon with rice, broccoli, carrots, and a salad. When a magazine writer asked her to name her five favorite foods, she said: "Pizza, pizza, pizza, pizza, and pizza." She does eat pizza on special occasions, but certainly not before a meet.

Biles knows the importance of rest and recovery. Since she doesn't have time for a nap, she makes sure to get at least eight hours of sleep each night. She gets up every morning by 7:45 am. For recovery after a workout, sometimes she wears compression pants to help increase blood flow and decrease recovery time. Other times she uses battery-powered boots that form around her legs and pulse air to provide a massage-like treatment.

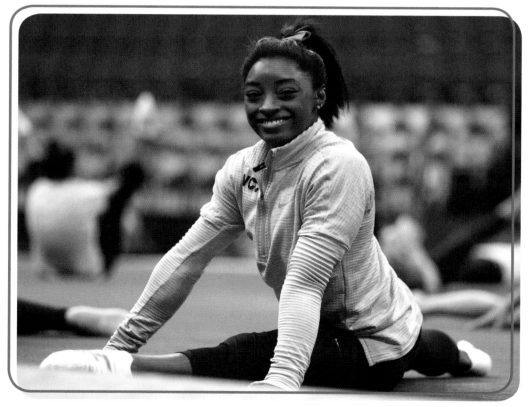

Biles knows the importance of stretching to keep her muscles warm and flexible.

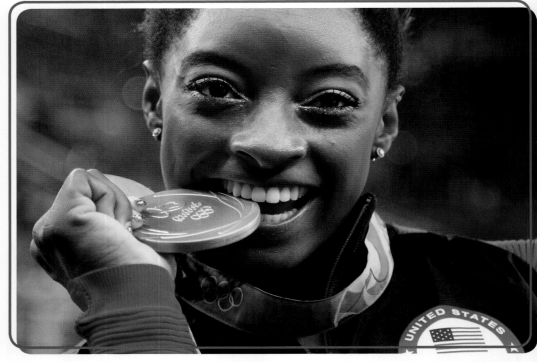

Nothing tastes sweeter than smart nutrition for Biles,
seen here savoring her Olympic gold medal win.

No other sport requires more mental strength than
gymnastics. What is mental strength? Imagine a
basketball player stepping to the free throw line to either
win or lose a game. All eyes are on the shooter—and he
or she knows it. The pressure can be unbearable. That's
what gymnasts feel—all the time. They stand alone and
try to be perfect. Their performance is greatly determined
by their mental strength.

In Biles's first senior national meet in 2013, she performed well below her ability. Her mother hired a sports psychologist to help her manage her nerves. Biles revealed her fears, her anxiety, and the pressure of potential failure. She learned coping techniques. She says her favorite competition ever was winning the 2013 Worlds because no one knew her, so she felt no pressure. After she won the 2015 Worlds, she only felt relief that it was over. The stress of being "unbeatable" was heavy. "I feel like I over think," she has explained many times to reporters. "As an event comes closer, even if I've hit sets for months, I'm like 'I can't do it anymore!' It's a habit that I've had for years and it hasn't stopped yet. I have to focus on not thinking." Just like training her body, now she is constantly training her mind.

Fun Fact

As a child, Simone was quite short for her age. "Growing up it was kind of a struggle being small since everyone would make fun of you," she says. "Except for when it came to play hide and seek— that's the only advantage I ever had!"

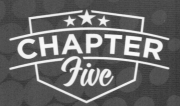

CHAPTER
Five

COMMITMENT

Biles rests on Sundays. She attends church, hangs out with friends at the Woodland Mall, and enjoys the family dinner. She is a superhero to most, but at home she is simply Simone. "My mom said it best, that 'We can be your family or your fans, but not both,'" brother Adam explained to a reporter. "We're her biggest supporters, but we don't go goo-goo and ga-ga. We keep it normal." The Biles family was recently asked to star in a reality TV series. They declined.

One way Biles manages pressure is to take an extra day off. She might ask to skip a Saturday practice. Beneath the costumes and ribbons is an intensely demanding sport—and missing training for two straight days is considered a long break. Biles is certainly driven to win for her team and for herself. But she knows best how to manage herself.

"I am confident that my coaches and I have found a system that best fits what my mind and body need in order for me to reach my goals," Biles told a reporter. "A lot of people compare me to other gymnasts. I don't want to replicate others. It's a matter of wanting to be the best version of me. I just want to go out there and be Simone."

Fun Fact

Biles is teamed up with Girls on the Run—an organization that promotes fitness for girls. Simone says: "I am who I am today because of sports. It has shaped me, taught me to become a leader and how to have confidence. I think sports and being physically active are very important for young girls."

AWARDS

U.S. all-around champion
5 times (2013, 2014, 2015, 2016, 2018)

World all-around champion
4 times (2013, 2014, 2015, 2018)

Women's Sports Foundation Sportswoman of the Year
(2014)

USOC's Female Athlete of the Year
(2014–15)

American record four Olympic gold medals
(2016)

Associated Press Female Athlete of the Year
(2016)

United States Sports Academy Female Athlete of the Year
(2016)

ESPNW's Woman of the Year
(2016)

Sports Illustrated's Fittest Female Athlete
(2017)

ESPY award—Best Female Athlete
(2017)

TIMELINE

1997 — born in Columbus, Ohio

2006 — enrolled in gymnastics

2008 — began training

2010 — first competition—Junior Olympic Level 10

2013 — won U.S. all-around title

2013 — won World all-around title

2014 — won U.S. all-around title

2014 — won World all-around title

2015 — graduated high school

2015 — won U.S. all-around title

2015 — won World all-around title

2016 — won four gold medals at Rio Olympics

2016 — set U.S. record with 19 total World/Olympic medals

2018 — won U.S. Classic

2018 — won both U.S. and World all-around titles

GLOSSARY

balance beam A long beam approximately four feet high and four inches wide

crunches A core exercise in which you lie on your back with your knees bent and feet flat on the floor and raise your upper body slightly off the floor while holding in your stomach

elite level The highest level of gymnastics

floor routine A series of dance and tumbling skills performed on a mat 40 feet long and wide

layout A position in which your body is completely stretched with your toes pointed straight

lunge A lower body exercise in which you step forward (or to one side) and lower yourself on one leg

pike A position in which your body is bent only at the hips

plank A core exercise in which you are in pushup position, except on your elbows

squat A lower body exercise starting from a standing position in which you bend your knees, as though seating yourself in a chair, and then stand back up

triathlon A multisport race in which you combine swimming, biking, and running without stopping

vault A bench-like table from which you push off with your arms to perform an aerobatic move

uneven bars Two parallel bars, approximately 5.4 feet and 8 feet in height

FURTHER READING

Dzidrums, Christine. *Simone Biles*. Whittier, CA: Creative Media, Inc, 2016.

Fishman, Jon. *Simone Biles*. Minneapolis: Lerner Publications, 2017.

Mattern, Joanne. *Simone Biles*. New York: Scholastic, 2017.

McAneney, Catie. *Simon Biles—Greatest Gymnast of All Time.* New York: Rosen Publishing, 2017.

ON THE INTERNET

www.simonebiles.com
Biles's official site

www.teamusa.org
The U.S. national team official site

www.usagym.org
The USA Gymnastics official site

INDEX

Bannon's Gymnastix	9
Belgium	9
Belize	12
Biles, Adam	27
Biles, Adria	8
Biles, Nellie	8
Biles, Ron	8
Biles, Simone	
childhood	7, 8, 9, 25
fitness	14, 16, 17, 18, 19, 20, 21, 24, 25, 26, 27
mental strength	24, 25, 27
nutrition	22
popularity	26, 28
youth competition	9, 10, 25
Biles, Shanon	8
Boorman, Aimee	9
China	9
Columbus, Ohio	4, 8, 29
Dancing With the Stars	12
Hawaii	12
Landi, Laurent	17
London	12
Monte Carlo	12
Olympics—Rio	11, 12, 13, 14, 29
Olympics—Tokyo	12
Retton, Mary Lou	15
Scotland	9
Spring, Texas	8
Woodland Mall	26
World Champions Centre	16
World Gymnastics Championships	9

ABOUT the AUTHOR

Jeff Savage is the award-winning author of more than 200 books for young readers. A former sportswriter for the *San Diego Union-Tribune*, Jeff's books have been read by millions. Jeff lives with his wife, Nancy, sons Taylor and Bailey, and dogs Tunes, Coach, Ace, Champ, Tank, and Lexi (that's six!) in Folsom, California. Jeff learned everything about Simone in a recent interview, except how to perform a handstand.